Living
Against All Odds

Living
Against All Odds

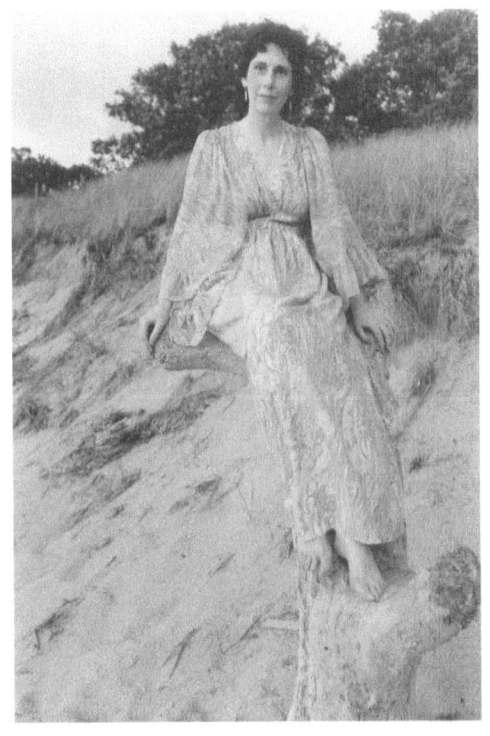

GERALD (JAY) GORDON

To order additional copies of this book, contact:
Xlibris Corporation
1-888-795-4274
www.Xlibris.com
Orders@Xlibris.com
67691

Contents

DEDICATED

TO THE MEMORY

OF

LOUISE HELEN ROEY GORDON

Louise cherished the immeasurable joy from her family and friends, to whom she was a strong support. Her love of life empowered her with a positive attitude in the face of medical obstacles. Louise did not see herself with physical limitations and as such, she remained an active participant in life. She would decorate her walker for festive occasions and roll off on her journey to traverse the architecturally and structurally difficult battlefield of twists and turns to experience the world. Her physician, attesting to her permanently disability, was in awe when she wanted to return to her job. "No" and "disabled" would never define Louise Gordon. Those words did not exist in her vocabulary. As her son Michael said, "She was intent on not spending her time dying, but intent on spending her time enjoying and living life. And live her life she did."

Louise Gordon's Medical History

(The short version in "layman's" terms)

Good health as child (usual childhood diseases) and young adult although I have taken Synthroid since I was 16 or 17. (Every physician I've seen since has tested to see if I really needed it. I do!)

1974   Appendix removed

1975   Gall Bladder removed

Early 1980s Arthroscopic knee surgery—right knee

1988   Tumor in T-11 discovered and removed. Diagnosis: Breast Cancer (no original site)

Three surgeries to try to biopsy and remove tumor and place Harrington Rods in my back while approximately 22 hours under anesthesia. Rods run from T-7 to L-3. Seventeen sessions of radiation to my back. In Michael Reese Hospital from February 8 to April 30.

Arthroscopic knee surgery—right knee.

1997   Soft tissue tumor found wound around spinal cord compressing it. Numb to waist by the time surgery commenced. 15 hours in surgery, but successfully removed. Diagnosis: Breast cancer. After one week sent to Rehabilitation Institute of Chicago. Returned to hospital where discovered I had developed antibodies to most of the antigens found in my blood. Hemolysis. Returned to rehab. Returned to hospital because of suspected infection in my back. Short 2-hour surgery to explore. Found Staph infection in my back, which was totally filled with pus. In ICU for 4 days while doctors try to figure out what to do. Hemolysis prevents the two 15-hour surgeries, neurosurgeon would need to remove and replace rods and totally clean out infection. Have 6-hour surgery to clean up back. Plastic surgeon cuts back muscle to bring blood supply and medication to parts of back needing the extra help. Prognosis: patient will not survive. I fooled them all. I'm still here! Entered Northwestern on 6-19-97 and left rehab on September 3rd. Trouble maintaining back in upright position, still partially numb in legs with some loss of balance.

2002   Still around to laugh. Back muscles will not support back in upright position and we have tried all sorts of physical therapy. I consider myself one hell of a lucky person!

Medicines 2/28/03

MEDICAL ALERT BRACELET—LEFT ARM

	Daily Amount	Amount/How Often
Aciphex	40 mg	20 mg twice a day
Amitriptylin	100 mg	100 mg at bedtime
Arimidex	1 mg	1 mg once a day
Atenolol	25 mg	25 mg once a day
Dicloxacill	2,000 mg	500 mg four times a day
Lipitor	10 mg	10 once a day
Oxybutynin	10 mg	5 mg twice a day
Synthroid	.25 mg	.25 mg once a day
Vioxx	50 mg	50 mg once a day

Ambien	10 mg	as needed
Alprazolam	.25 mg	as needed
Hydrocodone	5/500	as needed
Oxycontin	10 mg	as needed

Non-Prescriptions

Caltrate 600 + D		twice a day
Centrum Silver		evening
Vitamin E	400 I.U.	once a day

Louise Reflects

I am a cancer patient. I have been diagnosed as having metastasized breast cancer with no original site. The metastasis was located in T-11. As a result, I am being treated with Tamoxifen and undergo yearly mammograms and bone scans, along with seeing my oncologist 3 times a year, with a complete blood work-up each time.

Recently, I requested that we push up my bone scan because I felt "something funny" along my backbone. My oncologist agreed with me and suggested that I also have my mammogram at the same time. And so, I found myself having my usual screening tests within an 8-month interval. First, I received the results of my mammogram. There was something different about one area in my left breast. Yes, it had been there before, but . . . So, I was sent to a surgeon. He could see the area that they were talking about. He said that he wanted to have the radiologists at his medical center look at the films. If they felt that they could locate the area, then he would operate. He described the procedure as having a mammogram with a wire being used to locate the exact area. Then I would be brought to surgery to have the breast biopsy.

I became upset. Having been a part of a group at a Cancer Wellness Center, I had heard about this test. The comments I heard from women who had had this test was that it was very painful and that they could not understand why the doctors had not prepared them for the extent of pain. Okay, doctors! I realize that many women complain about the pain of a simple mammogram. And I realize that there is a local anesthetic used with this test. However, I do not understand how anyone could think that this would not be a *painful* test.

The surgeon assured me that only perhaps one patient a year complained about the pain to him—and he saw them right after the mammogram as he performed the breast biopsy with the wire in place to guide him. Maybe I was getting upset based on what people were saying and maybe they were wrong. So, I agreed that I would have the test and he agreed to give me Valium. Of course, I would have to wait to hear what the radiologists had to say.

I returned to work and became more upset. How could this test possibly not hurt? How deep does the anesthetic go? Would the whole area where the wire was inserted be numb? Wouldn't compressing the breast with a wire or needle inserted within the breast hurt?

That evening, I received a call from my oncologist telling me that the bone scan revealed some activity in the L4 and L5 area (just where I had complained of feeling funny). Therefore, he and I made arrangements to messenger the films of the most recent bone scan and at least one previous one to my surgeon. He also agreed to fax a copy of the reports (I go to the kind of doctors who believe that it is all right for me to know what is happening to my body. Yea!) to me at work.

The next morning, I called the orthopedist's office and made an appointment for the next available workday. As I was making this phone call on a Friday, this meant I would see the orthopedist on Monday. I also received a phone call from the surgeon who explained that the radiologists saw no reason to do a breast biopsy. This has left me with a lot of time (the weekend) to consider what is going on with my body and how I reacted to each bit of news and how I feel. That is why I am writing this.

Potentially, there could be far more serious problems with the bone scan. It could be a compression fracture. It could be degeneration. However, remember that the bone scan was had within 8 months because I felt funny. This is the same feeling I had had with the area at T-11, which caused a bone scan and an MRI to be performed and we realized that we were dealing with some type of growth, which was pushing my spinal cord. Hence, I had surgery to remove the tumor and to bolster the spinal column with rods, etc.

So why was I not crying and upset about the bone scan results and the potential for problems? This was the reaction I had to the wire mammogram. Why the difference in behavior?

My immediate reaction to that question is that there is something about the test and the reaction had by doctors that leaves me in tears. I do consider the test barbaric. But it is also necessary. However, I think it would help if a doctor would tell me that it is probably very uncomfortable and may be painful and, therefore, local anesthetic would be used generously and I would also receive tranquilizers which would make the whole procedure far easier to take. Now remember that I was told I could be given Valium, but that was only after I became visibly upset.

Louise's Life's Journey

The year was 1939. The continent, U.S.A. The city, New York's Bronx. The street, Bensonhurst. A young couple, Jacob (George) and Ethel Roey were blessed with their first born, Louise Helen Roey on February 17, of that year. Thus began her life's journey.

As with any parents, Ethel and Jacob gave a great deal of time and energy seeing to Louise's needs. Years passed as Louise flourished in their care. One plus and very positive side for Louise would be the fact that relatives lived only several blocks away. Therefore, it was no trouble to simply pop in, jump in and help and chitchat. Visits to and from the other families thus introduced Louise to an extremely important tenet in her life. Family! Family! Family!

Jacob was a successful lawyer who had many clients, both in and out of state. As time and demands increased, he was forced to move his family and household. After two such moves, Louise experienced the "new kid" syndrome. One of her dad's clients was NASA. Jacob was hired as inspector general to follow quality control, etc., for suppliers.

Louise entered the University of Massachusetts at the time her parents lived in Natick. Sophomore year at the university proved to be more interesting then academics. Louise met a young man in her classes. Her interest blossomed into love. She and the young man were engaged to wed. Unfortunately, he called it off and Louise was shattered. The only grace in the situation was that she was home on school break. Ethel and Jacob tried to console her and inasmuch as Louise loved board games, she and her parents played Monopoly into the wee hours of the mornings. Although the day brought a pressing schedule, nothing was more important then Louise. For, after all, nothing was more important than Family! Family! Family! How close can it get? Louise went on to get her degree.

After graduation, Louise was introduced to Arney. He was a Jewish lawyer who had completed studies on taxation while acing his Harvard exams. His prowess proved to be just that when he was hired by the IRS. It was said that Arney was one of three who knew all the ins and outs. By the way, he and Louise married and had three children: Miriam, born August 22, 1963; Phyllis, born March 24, 1965; and, Michael, born December 13, 1967. Louise taught 5th grade at Bradbury Heights Elementary School in 1961 and '62.

Arney moved his clan to Illinois where he joined a law firm located in the downtown ("Loop") area of Chicago. The couple purchased a townhome unit in Evanston, but all was not roses. Travel to Europe was no solution, nor did marriage counseling prove to be the answer. They filed for divorce. Arney moved to a Lakeshore Drive high-rise apartment, while Louise stayed in the home with the three children. She plunged into social activities, one of which was Amuse Register. Amuse was an adult camp located in Saugatuck, Michigan, which was operated by Presbyterians. Cabins, food and activities were provided for the week. It was not cheap and there was a long waiting list.

I was divorced "with custody" of my son, David. My plan was to drop him off at Evergreen College, located near Seattle, handle his college expenses and then continue on to L.A. Culver City as their manager. My plan was to begin a new life in the land of sunshine and oranges. I had been dating Elaine, a girlfriend of Louise's. Elaine had asked that I be added to the Amuse waiting list. The wheels of predestination spun into high gear and camp began. Louise's gentleman friend from a prior year was not interested and Elaine went on her way. Louise and I found common interests in consoling each other with respect to our similar losses. The week went by quickly, thus, it ended too soon. She had invited me to her home. When I arrived, there was a group socializing already and the place was wall-to-wall people. It seemed none wanted to miss any opportunity to be in the company of this charming, creative woman. When the crowd dispersed, I was invited to spend the night. David came with my pre-packed car. I kissed Louise "goodbye" and went to the trunk of the car where I retrieved a prize possession, a matched set of wood shaft golf clubs. I asked Louise to keep them, as she had not seen the last of me. I would be back!

How true those words became. As my son and I journeyed to L.A., there were more than food and pit stops; there were calls to Evanston, which became a constant. Yes, I had been bitten by the love bug. There were letters and telephone calls several times a day. After eight months, I asked Louise to marry me. She said, "Yes." I called the company's Chicago office and spoke to the vice president, Sol, about my leaving L.A. and returning to work for the company in Chicago. He said, "So you are getting married. Is she a great gal?" I replied, "Yes, Sol, she certainly is that and she has three children." Sol blew up and said, "Are you nuts?" I said, "Yes, Sol, I am. Love does that to you. The next big questions, is, can you find a spot for me in the organization?" Sol said, "Jay, for the years and dedication you have given Globe Glass, we need you." Arrangements were made for my L.A. replacement. I was going to Chicago! I called Louise and gave her the happy news and then I deadheaded to her home in Evanston, Illinois. I was now about to commence what I considered my second life.

It took me two days to drive from L.A. to Evanston. Louise and I were married on May 21, 1976, in the rabbi's study at Beth Emet Temple. My in-laws, Ethel and Jacob, were in attendance. They offered to stay with the children while we had our honeymoon weekend at a local area hotel. We had a second floor couch that miraculously turned into a hide-a-bed with a Stearns & Foster mattress.

After our honeymoon, the realities of my relationship with the children were spelled out. I was not their father. He was Arney. I was Jay, Louise's husband. The hope of a two-way street of respect was proposed. The children raised the question, "Should we be torn between families on holidays?" We agreed on a unified plan. Arney was welcome at our table for all events—birthdays, Thanksgiving, etc.—true unifamily. So parenting and life began again for both of us. The children's education continued with high school, college and all were shared.

Early in our marriage stands out in my mind that Globe Glass had furnished me with a van for transportation to and fro at any assigned office. I came home and parked in the rear alongside our car. As was my custom, I was entering the front door when I glanced at the passenger door of the car. It was caved in. I raced to the kitchen and yelled, "Louise, are you okay? What happened?" She had no idea why I was asking, as she had not been aware that the car door was damaged. One's loved ones and people are important, material things are secondary. I was relieved that she was okay and I gave myself a mental pat on the back.

Our life had its ups and downs until 1988, when Louise was diagnosed with breast cancer with no original site having been determined. There was a tumor wrapped around her spine. Delicate skills were hand-in-hand in the operating room. This procedure took many hours, with chemo and radiation treatments to follow. I can only imagine the nightmare of discomfort with pain as her constant companion. She had been hooked up to a morphine drip which, fortunately for Louise, she was able to control. The doctors were aware of her spirit, and speaking of that, with Passover approaching, Louise asked the Michael Reese staff to utilize a dayroom so we could celebrate the holiday. A caterer brought the traditional foods. Somehow the word got out. CBS interviewed Louise for a human-interest story. (We have a tape.) The word went out about what was happening in the room down the hall and a couple of interns looked in. Food samples were eaten with relish, including the horseradish for the fish. One day I took the day off and prepared Louise's favorite chicken livers with mushroom and onions. Hospital food is not very good. We ate, repeating and laughing, "With liver you live," a private joke between us. The children could not even stand the smell of the delicacy.

How vivid is the memory of Louise coming home. There was a line of chairs and teams of people to assist up the stairs, through the kitchen, to a hospital bed set up in the front room. We had a screen to provide her some privacy. Time, medications, family and her strong will propelled her strength, and she was soon able to climb the stairs to our bedroom, but for her sake and safety, one person in front and another behind her. In the ensuing years, we did everything. Louise's lust for life, her eyes viewed the ordinary as extraordinary. She was involved in ME (marriage encounter) group, as well as a women's support group. Her job, her family and religion gave support to her life. We didn't sit on the sidelines. Any aid, whether from walkers or other equipment, was adorned with flags and sometimes flowers. Louise's strength improved and slowly she was able to drive and return to work. We were proud to attend and be active parts of all three children's weddings. Her cancer didn't completely leave her body. Ten years afterward, in 1999, it reappeared on the original site of the spine, T-11. The surgery was performed at Northwestern Memorial Hospital. There were complications with strep throughout the entire spine. The doctors had to work around, but could not do the entire clean up. The blood plasma she received created antibodies so she was faced with yet another hurdle to overcome. Louise's life hung in the balance. A colleague at Northwestern University, where Louise worked, overheard her husband, who was a member of the team of Louise's doctors, say that it did not look good. The congregation of our temple prayed for her complete recovery, so there were many tears of many denominations in the mix, or at least I like to think so.

Many months later we brought Louise home with tears and joy. In the latter part of 2000, Louise and I traveled to Alaska on a cruise—a trip of a lifetime. We purchased a Toyota van which provided her with more ease and comfort getting in and out of her vehicle. Louise continued to work at Northwestern University's Development Office. To her, each day was a gift. My bride retired in February 2004. The retirement plans of travel were ended when she developed a cough that lingered for months. The cough did not stop her. Her doctor admitted her to Northwestern Memorial Hospital in early August 2004. After extensive examinations, the cancer was found throughout her lungs. On August 10, a Monday, we were at her bedside, for her and for each other, when the life sounds ended. Louise had given so much to all.

Dear Heart, you wanted to measure up to your idol of women of importance—Eleanor Roosevelt and Golda Meir. To me and many others, you continue to outshine them.

As always, my love,
Jay

Our heart is an organ
When we open our eyes
To humming birds, flowers, trees and sun
We can hear one heck, one heck of a song.
Louise, your heart played an unforgettable melody.

Louise's memories of the good times

We were married in May 1976. We met during the summer of 1975. When you moved to California in September 1975, you called me every day. So, even before we learned to love each other, I was fortunate enough to experience the soft, giving, caring side of you. Not only did we talk every night, but we also wrote letters to each other and we grew closer. When Phyllis had tests at Children's Memorial for a suspected brain tumor, you were there across the miles for me. And I felt loved and cared about, and, more important, not alone. You were also there when my father had his heart attack. Although you were many miles away, your caring and concern wrapped me up in a polar fleece blanket. Warm, light, soft and not suffocating.

I also have a picture of you sitting in our old blue chair, with Michael upon your lap. Even my mother, who was visiting at the time, saw your gentle, loving side as you interacted with Michael.

Throughout our marriage we shared many wonderful times. We shared many trips to my parents as well as many trips with them. I remember our second cruise with them. It was the beginning of the renewed relationship between my parents and my brother Hal and his wife Nan. We were the buffer zone, literally, between them. Our stateroom was the middle one between Hal and Nan's and my parents' cabin. Although Nan and Hal went off a lot on their own, we stayed with my parents most of the time; but we managed to find time for just the two of us also. We had so much fun together. But more than that, you enabled me to enjoy both you and my parents. All six of us had such a nice party for Dad's 80th birthday in our stateroom. We had snacks and champagne. Actually, the whole trip was delightful—with no housekeeping, dishes, or cooking. Just time for fun.

Our trip to Israel was a very special time. We met my parents in New York and flew to Israel in the same plane with them. We also spent some of the first week in Jerusalem with them. Then we went on our tour and they attended their Hadassah convention. We traveled through much of the country with other Americans and a delightful Israeli guide and bus driver. We were exposed to both the history and present-day Israel. That was a great education, reinforcing the history and politics of a country that was a part of my life from before the time I listened on the radio to the UN vote as they decided to partition Palestine. Pushing you along the cobblestones of Old Jerusalem in the wheelchair was not quite as hard as we shared the sights together. And I felt so close to you.

Sometime in our marriage I had an unusual experience. One night I dreamt of our having a little boy. I remember that the dream involved being pregnant and giving birth (it was obviously the easiest labor I had). When the little boy was born, he had a shock of black hair. We decided to name him after an uncle of mine who had died just a few years before. When I awoke, it was morning and Mother's Day. Your present to me was a little statue of a boy and his dog, running. We had decided not to have any children together when we first married. Maybe this expressed my desire to have a child with you. Anyway, the memory of the dream and sharing those feelings with you have always left me with such a good magical memory. Although we've not actually had a child together, we shared the dream, and the present, and the memory.

I don't even remember when one of our "no destination" vacations took place, but it was fun and provided me with more memories. We had no destination in mind, but we had a weekend with no children. We drove north, taking small roads, often choosing to go in any direction, whatever mood struck us. We even found ourselves circling around a couple of times, driving past an area we had driven past before, although not necessarily going in the same direction. After five hours of driving, we found ourselves in Kenosha, Wisconsin, and we stayed in a motel at the corner of 94 and route 50. I enjoyed our time together and the lack of structure. And we giggled at how long it took us to a place that was only an hour away from home.

How about the vacation where we made believe we were tourists. One day we took a red, double-decker bus through downtown Chicago. We broke up the bus trip and took a boat out on the lake, traveling up and down the lakeshore and up and down a short part of the river. Another day we went to the Museum of Science and Industry and took in the movie. Before the movie, we saw a few of the exhibits. Another time I remember we woke up late and you just wanted to watch the Cubs on television. We did that—totally unplanned and just a day of relaxing. Another time we went out for dinner and a movie. None of these things were extraordinary, but they were fun as we shared the time and the sights together as well as the lack of structure.

Another fun memory was buying a new car and trading in your old brown, second-hand one. I had to hide my face behind a newspaper as you bargained with the salesman. We were worried that the car would not start when they tried it, let alone that it was worth anything. It did start and we did trade it in for an air-conditioned Chevy Malibu wagon. That old brown car was the last non-air conditioned car we owned.

Have I told you how much I have enjoyed our trips to Iowa City to see my aunt and uncle? Jay, I enjoy visiting with them and when their old age gets to me, I realize that you and I aren't so far behind. But I do enjoy our trips. They are very low-keyed and relaxing and although we spend lots of time with my relatives, we also stay in a motel and have time for ourselves. My aunt and uncle are interesting people and I gain from touching base with my roots in the little way I can. I appreciate so much that you have not complained and have seemed to enjoy these visits also. Thank you.

It hasn't been only vacations that have given us the special moments that create the extra warm feelings for you. Sometime it has been an evening we've spent alone together. Sometimes we've rented a movie or two. Maybe it was a time of sharing a television show. It doesn't matter what we do. What matters are the feelings that are generated.

Recently, we've experienced the move to our new home. What pleasure we've had. I love living here. Life is so much easier. And this is the first home that we've shared that was "ours" from the beginning. To add to that, we are slowly furnishing it in a way to make our life and our lifestyle easier. Planning everything, choosing everything, anticipating and then living with what we've picked gives me so many positive feelings as we share each stage. We've spent so many joyful hours and days and there's still more to come.

And we've certainly had many delightful times with Selena. Just recently when we went to pick her up, you waited in the car and I went into Miriam and Ken's home to get her as we usually do. When we came outside, she ran ahead towards you calling, "Pop-Pop! I've missed you." Jay, how do we measure those kinds of memories? And they have been ours to share. That scene is perhaps even more meaningful to me because of Miriam telling me when she was pregnant, that you would not be her baby's grandfather. A month or two ago, before the above-mentioned scene with Selena, Miriam told me that you were Selena' s grandfather. That Selena could not love you more. Then this scene of this little 3-year-old running, with her long red hair flying behind her and her arms outstretched towards you. Jay, that kind of memory stirs up so much love and good feelings towards you from me.

We struggle together to live and share a lifetime. We are different and we expect different things from a marriage. Some chasms we will never fill in. Writing about positive events, sharing good memories, this is what makes the difficult times not so difficult. Jay, we have so many good memories together that it is sometimes hard to remember them all. But it's those memories and many more that help us through life and make the rough times easier to deal with.

We aren't that old, but we are growing older. I see both of us slipping in many ways. And it is scary. But those memories, hopefully, will help us use our love to pull us through some of the difficult times that are with us now and those that will be in our future. It will be much easier to face them together.

I love you,
Louise

Reflections

One thing that stands out where I think of my mother is that she found happiness in the little things. I remember her driving and pointing out the flowers, trees, clouds and noticing their beauty. I remember thinking it was silly, even corny. But, as I've gotten older, I find myself doing the same thing—noticing the beauty in the little, everyday things. And I find myself pointing out these same things to my daughter, hoping that she will learn the same things that I did from my mother.

Phyllis Cohen-Marshall

Louise, If You Please

Take our Louise, if you please.
But not too far—perhaps to another star.

Give her new voice, so others can rejoice
At her message so clear, all can adhere.

A woman who loved life, who was a good wife.
Devoted to children three, and theirs also to a high degree.

A steady friend as the need arises, at that there's no surprises.
Offering help and good advice, your benefit is the only price.

Responsible to jobs varied, unexpected burdens easily carried.
Adaptable, flexible and caring, co-workers valued her sharing.

Think of determination and grit—that lady is it.
What she wanted to do was likely to come true.

Life issues and adversity, she met with great dignity.
That's our Louise, if you please.

With love, Alan Friedlander

Dear Jay,

When Louise crossed over the rainbow, we lost a great couple. For without Louise, there was no way for you to comfortably continue in our marriage encounter group. Our loss was doubled by your absence.

Over our many years together we came to rely upon the Gordons to help spark our evenings together. We were never let down, even on the one occasion when you left your talk at home. Somehow the two of you held together and provided us with a very special ME evening.

Your Louise was a very special lady. Her smile alone could light up a room and often did. Her physical limitations from cancer surgery never seemed to get her down, certainly not in the presence of our ME group. She, like Proud Mary, just kept rolling along, with everyone else following in her wake, gladly!

On the several occasions we visited Louise in the hospital, she was the one to lift up our spirits, not the other way around. Some gal, that Louise.

Who can forget her running countdown to her retirement? It became a standing joke to hear her recite years, months, days, hours, and even minutes, to her long-awaited days of leisure. She planned everything, or so it seemed. Moving into the condo, getting a dog, where to go, what to do, family, friends to see. She was full of positives for the possibilities of life, and there was Jay, along for the ride of his life at the side of his very special lady.

She is missed, you are missed, but never forgotten. You betcha!!.

Love,
Cliff and Freddi Krell

A *letter about Louise* ...

When Jay phoned and asked me to write a few words about my friendship with Louise, I jumped at the opportunity and believed that I would just whip something out in the following few days . . . . or so I thought! Days turned into weeks and the notion of actually writing my thoughts down became a real challenge, because I wanted to get it right!

After the second call from Jay, I told myself that it would not be easy to write just a few words to describe such a long-term friendship, but I had to try again . . . . and right away!

Our "sisterhood" was formed many years before I joined it. I was the "newby" having met the Group for the first time at a bridal shower for Joan Lawson whom I had met through a women's business group in Crystal Lake. I could tell that I was being sized up, and, much to my surprise, was invited soon thereafter to come to one of the meetings of the Group! That was almost twenty-five years ago!

The drive for me was about twenty-five miles each way, and meeting every two weeks was a strain, but I kept going. There was something about this group that I liked, and I wanted more of it! There were six members including me . . . . and there couldn't have been greater diversity amongst us! We had different backgrounds; we didn't look *anything* alike; our ages were all over the board beginning with the baby of the Group in her 30s and the oldest in her 60s; but, each had something different to offer the Group. We began calling ourselves "sisters"! A couple of times during a year, the Group would go somewhere for the weekend, and fun we had!

So many laughs and a few tears shed along the way. What great therapy, though, from a group of women whose friendship you knew you could trust! No one else, though, actually believed that we were sisters!

Louise had been through a lot . . . . serious surgeries and rehabilitations. She showed strength of character and enthusiasm for the future which I don't think many others in similar circumstances have. Always appreciative of her faith, family and friends, I never heard her even whisper a word of unkindness about anyone! Every time that there was a good result from a medical test for her to report to the Group, everyone would be enormously relieved and happy!

The Group still meets, though very irregularly, but it will never be the same without our dear Louise . . . .

Still missing my friend,
Judith Sedlack

June 10, 1997

Dear Roberta and Wally:

After a long draught and not being in touch, a letter is easier for me. It's very difficult to realize how long the time has been since I've been in touch with you.

On the good side of life, I am working as a secretary in the Office of Development at Northwestern University. I enjoy the work and the people with whom I work could not be nicer or more wonderful. Jay is working 12 hours a week with LifeSource (the blood bank—I always knew there was a dark side to him) and delivering meals one day a week to the elderly. My almost 2-year-old granddaughter (Miriam and Ken's) Selena is an absolute joy who gives me a shot in the arm of love, peace and the continuation of life. She is, of course, perfect in every way; however, since her humming consists of a one note tone no matter what she is humming, I do not think she will make it in the singing field. Selena usually spends Saturdays with us and loves playing with Sesame Street computer programs as well as other programs geared to her age. I get a little bored with what entertains her, but she thinks the only way she can play with the computer is to sit on my lap—and to hold her is like the whipped cream on the top of a marvelous dessert. I am also the grandmother of a 12-week-old kitten, (Phyllis') Pepper,—the name suggestion was Ken's since she is black with some white hairs scattered about). Pepper brings company to Phyllis and she loves coming to our house. In fact, to make it easier for Phyllis to visit us more often (she can't leave the cat alone too much), we are going to accept a litter box, food and water dishes and everything that goes into them! That probably should have been put into the section entitled "challenges" which follows, but then again, the lilt in Phyllis' voice definitely adds Pepper to the "good side of life."

On the challenging side of life, my cancer has returned. Actually, the numbers in a blood test have been going up and up for over two years, although we have not been able to locate it primarily because MRIs cannot be taken of my back because of the rods. Just recently, with the second neurologist, we have discovered a soft-tissue mass at the same location as the first site—T-II. This time, it is wrapped around the spinal cord and is compressing the cord. It will take unusual skill to be able to remove it without hurting the spinal cord. There are 3 rods in that area, removing all hope of moving the vertebrae in order to get to different areas of the spine. I've been using a walker for several months since my legs are numb and I do not have good balance any more. Right now I am hoping that we will schedule the necessary surgery and get on with life. I'm sure that I'll finally be one of the many who is on chemo after all of this—so I am hopeful.

Louise

September 1998

Dear Louise:

Our eyes are looking toward tomorrow and the future while our backs are warmed by the yesterdays of 22 plus years of marriage. I can recall so many bright moments so why don't I start with our wedding day. Your folks came in from Florida with a pronouncement that they were prepared to stay with us for a second week so they could watch the kids the following weekend. We gratefully accepted their gift of time and made a reservation at Shangri-La Howard Johnson—the place for newly weds on Skokie Boulevard. What more could a couple need: food—Don's Market—, a swimming pool and, most of all, privacy. We spent a night of hugs, snacks and togetherness that continued to the wee hours of the morning. We were watching color TV, which stopped broadcasting and we were watching black and white.

In December 1983, we gave your folks a 50th anniversary party in a hotel in Florida. It was a monumental task that took on many of the decisions of an actual wedding: the preparations, menus, invitations, location, wine, music, photographer, wedding cake, etc. Honey, you did it. I was shaking in my boots. Could we pull this off? The role of host was one I was not comfortable assuming. The hit of the evening was when your parents sat side-by-side while a ceremony took place acknowledging their togetherness and love. It was lovely. Although the role of host was unfamiliar, you prompted me on the amount to be tipped for various services. I felt like a big shot. I felt close to you and was filled with hope that we would be lucky enough to enjoy our years together as your parents enjoyed their years together.

Many years later we had another wonderful idea. Why not visit Israel? Our Rabbi's wife is a travel agent who would certainly see to our special needs of my limited mobility. A tour group, transportation, hotels, airline (what else? El Al!) and points of interest were all arranged. We got into high gear for our part. There were passports, travelers' checks, clothing and rolls of film. We were told that should be a difficult item to obtain in Israel. Well, you know we bought more than one and less than a thousand—20 rolls as I recall. We arrived at Ben Gurion Airport and landed away from the building. Large buses picked us up to take us to the terminal. This was standard; however, I found it unusual. The days that followed were filled with sights: The Wall, Temples, archeological digs, Messada and the local market with merchandise, food, spices and everything imaginable. Our home base while in Jerusalem was a fine hotel, clean, good food and fine service. At one of our meals, the waitress came to our table while we were engrossed in conversation and asked us in Hebrew what we wanted to order. We explained we were Americans who did not speak Hebrew. The waitress apologized for having mistaken us for natives. The rich heritage of our people filled me with pride. I soared as the birds from Messada's Heights.

Recently, after a busy weekend, we prepared for bed rather late. Your Monday morning comes around very early. As is the case many nights, you weren't able to sleep, so off to the computer room you went. That often lulls you to sleep. Your alarm went off shortly after 6 a.m. Turning, I realized you weren't in bed. This was unusual, so I jumped up to see where you were and if everything was all right. You weren't in the bathroom, nor were you in the computer room. I walked into the living room. There you were stretched out on the couch, covered with a throw. Waiting for a few minutes, I sat down in the chair along side of you with an eye on the clock. I waited for you to awaken. At 6:30, I stroked your arm gently. This may sound strange, but when you awakened with a smile and a thank you, there was a moment of realization of how deeply I cared and how much I love you. The old Ralph Kramden quote, "How sweet it is," hit home.

How quickly time has passed. It's been a little over 3 years since Selena was born. Miriam told you while she was pregnant that there was no way that I could be considered Selena's grandfather. Time has passed with the little one letting us know who is boss. She has let her mother know that her Pop-Pop is important in spite of the lack of biological connection. When we picked up Selena recently, she ran down the stairs with her hands out, shouting, "Pop-Pop, I missed you." I bent down and picked her up in my arms and hugged and kissed her. What a wonderful, unsolicited gift. I felt humble and elated to have all that love.

When night falls, we are able to see many stars. However, when I close my eyes, the sky reflects the many special memories we've shared.

With love,
Jay

In Memory of Louise R. Gordon

When two lives touch, they can never really be separated

Have you ever imagined the fright experienced by a writer when he encounters his first blank page, or an artist contemplating a canvas? As both, I can tell you it is simply overwhelming. However, if you can imagine that, then you may have some under-standing of what one's life would be like without Louise Gordon in it. Blank! Empty! Stark-naked, void, depleted, desolate, shallow, dark, dank, thin, wasted, hollow, vacant, discarded, cancelled, invalid, negated, gloomy, dismal, austere, and bleak, too! That is overwhelming. Now let me take you to the brighter side of the written page and the painted canvas and introduce you to a woman who would disagree with every adjective used thus far. The perpetual optimist . . . . my friend, Louise.

If the years before meeting Louise Gordon had been a blessing of which I was never aware, then those that followed my introduction to her were definitely a joy and a true gift from God. Everyday life before meeting Louise was simply okay; but after meeting her, it became an inspiring experience. Each day brought with it new awakenings, new discussions and resolutions, which often came out of reflections of the past where it was acceptable to visit but never acceptable to stay too long. Over the 30+ years that I had lived in the Chicago-Skokie-Evanston area, I managed to keep as many people at arm's length as possible. Then Louise (and Jay . . . . let's not discount Jay) came into my life and therewith came the realization that there are really some very admirable people in this world—and some of them never make the headlines or the 5:00 o'clock news, nor do they get the recognition they ultimately deserve. Louise and Jay were two such people. It has been eleven years since I moved into the Enclave, so rationally speaking, that means I met Louise sometime in very early 1998. I have absolutely no recollection of the circumstances of our first meeting but I can share with you that I was not the same after meeting her.

Come along on a journey with me and picture, if you will, a woman who was the exact opposite of each and every adjective used above. There are round words like Ohio, balloon, oval, apple and elliptical, which, although not round, fits in its circular family. There are long words like river, winding, Long Island, Mississippi, Pennsylvania, trail and train, which, although it contains few letters, can be very lengthy, drawn out and seemingly unending, adding some length of its own. There are short words like rope, which can be a terribly long word, too. There is "little" which is anything but short with its four ascenders. There are deep words like cellar, basement, quicksand, mind, oil well and ocean, which is round, and wet, as well. But hole, a deep abyss, while round, should never be confused with whole, which is thorough and all-encompassing. Words like slim, elevator, slender, escalator, windmill and stairwell speak to heights. There are words that speak to shapes such as pear, square and legs, which, if you will, are slightly more shapely than narrow. Don't forget liquid, which, in reality, has a myriad of shapes.

As words go, there are many which I find to be descriptive of my dear friend, Louise. Just as liquid flows when out of its container, so went Louise Gordon. She went anywhere and everywhere she could. She had a will to prevail. Louise was always attempting to make everything easier and not just because of her medical issues. She made things more convenient and accessible for everyone. No matter how many times I had offered any kind of physical assistance, whether that was opening a door, holding a door or taking something from her walker, about the only help she would accept was my closing the van door after she was in as we would prepare to leave for work. For a long stretch of time, Louise gave me a ride to work in the mornings even though that drive took her blocks out of her way. She knew I often took the bus home which meant I had a 20-minute walk from the seminary to downtown Evanston. We started our workday at the same time, but I finished at 4:30. If it was raining or snowing, Louise would call and say, "I can't leave until 5 as you know, but stay there because I'm coming to pick you up. No need for you to walk in this mess or to get wet." And "no" was not an acceptable answer from me. She was a headstrong woman who made decisions based on what she felt was right and just. I think we both had similar definitions of sympathy—that being, if you were looking for it in us, it was there, but only after you tried all the possible alternatives. Louise didn't feel sorry for herself. She accepted the cards that life dealt to her for what they were, but she did her levelheaded best to circumnavigate whatever the challenge was. She looked at them head on, accepted whatever it was, decided how she would deal with it, and then proceeded to live her life with and through it.

Selecting one word that is most descriptive of her is difficult to discern. Three come to mind. The first, **inclusive**—because she brought you out of yourself and into a world that introduced you to life and living it. The second, and perhaps the better choice of these two—**encompassing**—as she expanded the circumference of every descriptive adjective and noun in any dictionary. She not only offered you her hand, she offered you her heart. Anyone who experienced Louise in his or her life had a friend for life. Just look around. She's still with you. You cannot see her, but you can talk to her. As for those individuals nearby who might think you are talking to yourself, well, you know Louise would have a good laugh looking at their puzzled faces as they watch you talking to yourself. The third word, **THERE**, probably seems a weird and strange choice and hardly descriptive of the person you might have known. But there it is! My final selection that describes Louise Gordon to the fullest. She was always there. Just there! Her constant was "THERE" although I am not sure she knew it. When you called her to ask how she was, she was there, but instead she wanted to talk about how you were. When you called to share your troubles and concerns, wasn't she always there for you? When you needed a hand, or often didn't think you did, wasn't hers always the one you found right there along side of your own. If one considers the definition of 'there," meaning "in or at that place where *you* are," then you know where you could always find Louise. Wherever *you* were. If she was not with you, in her physical form, you knew you could always find her in your heart as well as in your mind. She was one of those rare commodities that was always with you. Right THERE! Just THERE!

"There! It's done," is an exclamation used to express satisfaction, relief, encouragement, consolation and the like. I am very satisfied with my dear friend. I am relieved and honored to have had her in my life. She shared with me both her encouragement and her consolation, as well as her wisdom, laughter, and above all, her love for people and her love of life in spite of what fate dealt us. I knew I had a place in her heart that belonged only to me . . . we all had our own special place in that huge heart. She would tell you what was what, and perhaps even more than you wanted to hear—and often her words came unsolicited. She simply cared enough to say what was on her mind.

Are there enough adjectives in a dictionary to describe this woman? Yes. Would she have been a strong candidate for Women's Rights? Yes. For anyone's rights? Most assuredly. Would she give you unsolicited advice? Yes. Why? Because she cared and please note that she didn't have to be very fond of anyone to care about them. Many years ago, having been raised Roman Catholic, I recall that the church published a monthly newspaper in which were listed all the current movies and each was listed under some specific heading. I always looked first at the ones under "Condemned" because I wanted to know which movies the church thought I should not see. Then I'd checked out those under "Objectionable in Part" for those would be the next ones on my list to see. Whenever someone told me or suggested to me that there was something I SHOULD NOT do, I would head for that venue instantly. Louise was one of those people whose personality defied anyone to tell her she could not do something and subsequently that personality was one to encourage others to investigate, to learn, to educate themselves in all the venues life had to offer. She often said to me, "The only thing that stops anyone from doing something is himself. We have a habit of getting in our own way." And she would add, "You don't have to do it all at once either. There is nothing wrong with taking it one step at a time. Learning goes on. It just doesn't stop once you have learned something. That learning leads to other avenues to be explored."

In sharing more beautiful, lovely, charming adjectives and heartwarming stories of Louise, I know firsthand of her kindness and thoughtful good nature. I have been a recipient of her benevolence, wisdom, caring, concern and love. In July 2004 I had my total left hip replacement surgery. We had talked about the surgery for months before the actual event. Louise called me at the hospital to see how I was doing. She was concerned. I was doing well and she said when I got into rehab she would come visit. Prior to my surgery she and I had many discussions about my rehab and what I should expect and to check out the places because I should go to a place where this, that and the other were all available. She had participated in a great deal of rehab as a result of her own medical problems and she knew what she was talking about. She wanted to make certain that I was going to have the kind of therapy that was going to restore me to full use of my leg. I recall the last time I saw my dear friend.

She came to visit me on a Sunday afternoon. It was very very hot in St. Francis Rehabilitation Center on Oakton and Dodge in Evanston. My room there was so insufferably hot, that I took up residence in the chapel. I probably would not have found that place save for the assistance of one of the chaplains who saw my distress and said, "Let me show you were the coldest place is in this building." I was amazed when she led me into the little chapel. Except for meals, that is where I spent most of my days and nights. It truly was the coolest place—in more ways than one. Louise and I sat for about an hour and just chatted. We got caught up on how things were going at the Enclave—one of our favorite topics of discussion. She told me that she was going to see her doctor the next day. We had our usual exchange of ideas and best wishes and she left for home. I left rehab on Wednesday and came home to learn that Louise's doctor had sent her on to the hospital and she was still there. On Friday, Louise called me from her hospital bed. She told me she had taken off the oxygen mask so she could talk to me. We had the usual discussions. "How are you? I'm fine. How are you? What does the doctor say? Oh let's not talk about me. How are you doing? Anything you need?" That was Louise! Always wanted to know how someone else was doing and what he or she needed. We agreed that we would rehab together when she returned home. We'd watch videos together, play board games, we'd saunter around the Enclave perimeter but only if it wasn't too hot. We never got to do those things we planned. Louise passed away in the hospital. I think it was not until I heard that news that I really thought about what an influence and force she had been in my life. She was one of the few people who realized that I was such a softie at heart, the one who hid behind the facade of a curmudgeon. She often said in those short rides to work, "If people knew the real you, the memory you have, they would be in awe."

And how many of us who knew Louise stood in awe of this woman who was a hands-on, in-charge lady whose life seemed to be lived around a three word phrase—"YES" and "I/You/We/They" and "CAN"? Yes you can. And she did! I think she must have always been a formidable force in all the lives she touched. One would hardly say or whisper, "I can't" in her presence simply because we all knew that if she heard it, she would ask, "Why not!" And there was never a question mark after her question. It always seemed to come with a big exclamation point, that punctuation mark that implies "action required"! I often wondered if she missed her calling and if she shouldn't have been a teacher.

I have many special memories of Louise that I will always cherish. My Monday through Friday drives to work over the last four years have reminded me every day of Louise as I travel the same route she traveled to work. We laughed and cried together. We talked for what seemed like hours about things important to both of us. We often talked about her cancer and her surgeries, the close calls with death and when she developed a tickling cough, I shared my concern. She told me it was just a touch of a cold according to her doctor, and later on, it was a cold that was hanging on. It was at a time when many people I knew were coming down with a similar problem that was diagnosed as a virus that was just taking its time. As months passed, it came time for Louise to retire from Northwestern's development office. The tickle persisted, but then so did Louise. She and Jay had purchased a van and then a powered vehicle (I called it the Enclave Dodgem) and she managed to get herself around with it. She was making plans for enlarging their unit entrance, and if necessary to have the lobby/garage door opening enlarged. Even though she retired in February of 2004, Louise still offered to drive me to work every morning, an offer I could not accept. She would call at 4:00 in the afternoon on rainy days to ask if I needed a ride home. In spite of my "No, but thank you for asking," she would come and get me. She had been most gracious and kind to me during the many months we did ride together but I certainly wasn't going to have her getting up early and dressing so she could drive me to work and I didn't want her coming out to pick me up at quitting time. I needed to rely on my own resources and she needed to become accustomed to being retired and enjoying it.

She never said she didn't have time. We even disagreed over many things. I experienced her ability to forgive and to forget and her willingness to repair. She and I did not always agree and there were some occasions when we were on the condo board together where that old adage of "seeing eye-to-eye" was nonexistent where we were concerned. It seemed to me that Louise was not confrontational—at least that was my perception. She was more or less just the opposite. She would state and defend her position and skillfully observed others state and defend theirs with the hope that once all was said and done, there was some sort of happy medium resolution. I wanted to encourage her to be more demonstrative in her approach, but she was a woman far wiser than I gave her credit for being initially. She always managed to get her point across. She was an admirable adversary and a substantial support to many.

She was a woman who was passionate about her adoring husband. She was not one to give up. I can recall only one time when she actually asked me for help. Jay was ill and she could not get him to take his medication and she could not lift him into a sitting position so she could make him take it. She called and of course, I went immediately. We got him to take his medication. Louise was very excited about getting a puppy. As she explained to me very early on, "I need to do this so Jay will have company when I'm gone." I started to ask what this "gone" business meant, but she overtalked me . . . or outtalked me, one or the other. For me that was her way of saying, "I've made up my mind and I'm not going to discuss it." I knew not to inquire further. She was also passionate about her children, their spouses and her grandchildren. She asked me once about framing the children's wedding photos so they could be displayed on the wall. We never got to complete that project. And every morning she had photos of the grandchildren to share on the ride to work, or she had stories of what they had done together or what she had planned to do with them during her retirement. She was very passionate about her family and the extended families and friends that comprised the Louise and Jay Gordon world.

Aren't we, her family and friends, the most fortunate to have the culmination of all words as one of our own? LOUISE! A woman of three special words—experienced deep in the hearts and minds of those with whom she had chosen to share them.

Since her passing, I have often reflected on the many wonderful years my friend had related to me about her life and how remarkable she made those years, not only for herself, but also for others, by giving of herself and by doing for others. In her last days, as sick as she was, she was still thinking of others. I truly believe that part of her legacy is her strong will, along with her faith in herself. Maybe even in a higher power. We never really talked about a higher power of any denomination. Just thinking back on so many wonderful memories of Louise, I am reminded that I still have a life to live—and not one that is reflected in mirrors and glass panes. Nor one that is enhanced by a colorful shirt or tie or jeans and sweater or fancy car, but rather one that is reflected in the eyes and hearts of those for whom we make life a better place. I cried like an innocent child at her service and yes, tears well in my eyes even now as I write this for her memorial book. But today I am not saddened by the short time we had together. Instead I rejoice that Louise Gordon came into my life and that we shared some time together. She enriched my heart, my soul and my mind. She was my very dear friend.

Ron Kucirko

Come, Sit Here With Me

It was a fall Friday night in 1993 when I timidly climbed the steps to the entrance of Beth Emet Synagogue in Evanston, Illinois. I was alone, a stranger to a new place and to a new people. I stood outside the main door, hesitating, ready to turn back and go home. No, the rabbi had said I was to begin attendance at Friday night services. This was my first time, after a year of studying with him, and after my mikvah immersion ceremony to seal my new identity as a Jew. I entered the main door and followed several people into the sanctuary, with a blue book handed to me by the usher. The sanctuary was filling up, people sitting or standing, the room abuzz with chatter and greetings, unseeing me. Where should I sit? There were vacant pews, but I gravitated to the back of the room where several rows, practically devoid of people, stretched across the back of the sanctuary. I stood with my back to the wall, trying to decide where to sit, preferably as far away from anyone as I could get. In the furthest back row a lone woman looked up at me, smiled, and in a melodious voice, called out, "Hello! Is this your first time here?" I stepped closer to her, smiled in return, and said, "Yes."

"Come," she said, "sit here with me." The sincere warmth and welcome in her voice and in her face were unmistakable. Gratefully, I stepped into the row of seats and sat next to her, near the aisle. "I'm Louise Gordon," she said, "Shabbat Shalom." "I am Barbara-Ann Lewis," I replied. "I have never been here before."

That was the first of many Friday nights for years, of sitting together, of coming early and sharing the week's happenings, of sharing the joys and sadness that come with families, of births and antics of grandchildren, anxieties of family and personal illnesses, of talking about the big questions of life and God. We sat together, too, during the long, somber day of Yom Kippur, and laughing over the incongruous actions of Rabbi Knobel and his Dov Bear during the children's services.

Louise guided me through the intricacies of the Friday night service and the prayer book with all its different parts. She predicted that I would learn all the Hebrew songs simply by coming every Friday night even if I didn't always know what they meant, just as she didn't always know what they meant. She pointed out specific people in the synagogue such as Sophie and Sid Black who were "very learned and very kind, the most important people at Beth Emet." I soon found out for myself that this was true, as were all of Louise's short commentaries on people she pointed out to me at the Friday night services.

I marveled at Louise's persistence in commuting to her daily job despite some pain due to past illness. She had good things to say about her co-workers, and matter-of-fact acceptance of those with less than stellar qualities. Her love for Jay, her husband, and her three grown children, Miriam, Phyllis, and Michael, was always evident. She had her time for "play"—occasional weekend outings with her group of 4 or 5 women friends that had been going on for a long time. She loved books and reading, and she loved Judaism. Her only discouragement was about herself and her lack of learning in Judaism. While she was growing up her parents, of blessed memory, did not think it appropriate or necessary for a girl to have much knowledge of Judaism. She mentioned boxes of her parents' books in her basement that she longed to read and understand. Since I was in the beginnings of Jewish knowledge myself, we shared what we knew with each other, and shared our longing to wear the "*tallit*" that signified to us, correctly or not, Jewish learnedness. When I began my studies to become Bat Mitzvah, not knowing if I would ever succeed, she decided that she would make the attempt herself, going beyond her parents' expectations for her. It took us about 2 years, but we did it.

Louise eventually changed jobs, cutting out her long commute by moving to the Development Office of Northwestern University. She enjoyed her work immensely despite increasing physical pain and despite occasional "difficult people." Her almost constant cheerfulness on Friday nights put my grumpiness to shame (I don't deal easily with "difficult people"), and quickly washed away the dross of the week and allowed me to immerse totally in Shabbat. Others sometimes sat with us, particularly Benjamin

Davidson, and Louise's cheerfulness spread even further. She loved the Friday evening services and hardly ever missed one, through darkness or cold. When I suggested that she try the Saturday morning services, she quickly let me know that her Saturday mornings belonged to Selena, her granddaughter, and later to Jacob her grandson, and nothing would change that.

Louise looked forward to retirement—she planned to volunteer at the Beth Emet Early Childhood program, and to take more Judaic courses in the evenings. She eventually did retire when her pain and surgeries made it impossible for her to continue working, nor was she able to carry out her retirement plans. As her pain increased, she continued to come to Friday night services as often as she could, and her bravery and cheerfulness through it all was an inspiration to me. She became quite bent over and needed to use a walker, but handled it often quite recklessly, often taking the down-ramp outside Beth Emet at break-neck speed, scaring me half to death. She would laugh when I accused her of being a terrible walker driver. She stubbornly refused what little help I could offer in loading and unloading the walker from her car. Stubbornness was a frustrating characteristic of Louise that I came to know and love over the years, and there were times, during her really bad pain when I believed that it was only her stubbornness that kept her going. She and Jay took at least one trip abroad, and she laughed while telling what it was like for two people with walkers to travel. She told me how grateful she was to Elaine Knobel who arranged their trips and made it all happen.

It was impossible for me to know the extent of her suffering, because she did not allow anything but cheerful, matter of fact words to talk about her condition to me. Even during our last conversation over the telephone as she lay in her hospital bed, she was perky and nonchalant—it was readily apparent that her main concern was not to cause me worry or grief. She forgot that where there is love, there will be grief.

It is said that seats at Beth Emet services are not reserved for anyone, but those seats in the back row belonged to Louise, Benjamin, and me. Now, it's only Benjamin and I who are often seen in the back row, but as far as I am concerned, Louise is there, too.

Barbara-Ann G. Lewis
21 April 2008

April 5, 2003

Dear Jay,

In my young adult life growing older did not mean becoming handicapped and facing some of the different problems. My mom had a prolapsed mitral valve with symptoms starting in 1947, when she was 37 years old. She died of congestive heart failure at the age of 78. I do not know if both of those were connected, but I had been watching her slowly become weaker as 1987 progressed. During the evening of February 19,1988, a day in which she had attended a class at the synagogue, she told my father she didn't feel well and he walked her to the bedroom and she lay down. Ten minutes later dad went to check on her and she was gone.

Dad had a heart attack and was in intensive care in June 1991. My brother called the doctor and was told dad would be fine and there was no need for him to rush to Florida. I didn't call and rushed down. I spent a week there and knew that my vacation days were getting slimmer, so we made arrangements for Michael to come down and take over for me. Michael arrived on June 7th and dad was moved to a step-down ICU. Dad had a heart attack and died that day.

During that last year of my mother's life, we went to Israel with Mom and Dad and to New Orleans with them along with my brother and sister-in-law. They lived a full and beautiful life. So why are we charged with supporting the medical community? Are we making up for the previous generations?

It took a long time from the time your internist told us your PSA had gone up and we received the results from the biopsy—you have prostate cancer. When I first heard the PSA was up, I thought it would be another false alarm as it was a few years ago. I felt this was just another scare and when it was all over, we would laugh at how the PSA blood test results just did not apply to you. When I heard it was cancer, I still did not feel it was that big a deal (well of course it wasn't—for me. I didn't have the cancer!). Prostate cancer, when caught early, usually responds to treatment and for many men, they are cancer free. But you seemed to be more upset about prostate cancer than the lung cancer you had in 2000. Following the initial lung surgery, you had more complications. Your nervousness about the prostate cancer did not add up. So what is going on with you? Is it because of the location of the cancer? Is it because you had such a rough time in 2000? Or perhaps is it because you didn't have options with the lung cancer and here you do?

There are 4 different ways to treat prostate cancer: 1) do nothing, just monitor it and hope that it is a very slow growing cancer; 2) surgery; 3) hormones; and 4) radiation. And within the radiation field there are two different ways to deal with that: traditional radiation and the planting of radioactive seeds in the prostate. We turned to our sources for information and everyone said radiation was the way to go, especially since the doctors felt you were not a good surgery candidate.

Finally, you confessed that you were very much afraid of the radiation. OK, I couldn't understand that, but at least I understood how you felt. For me, I knew that I had to keep my mouth shut. This had to be your decision. So my job is to give you love and support. This is hard for me—not the love and support part—but keeping my mouth shut. I have opinions about what I'd do if it were my body. Yes, I do feel as if invisible duct tape is covering my mouth. I want to shout out and scream—maybe have a full-scale temper tantrum. But you must make up your own mind. Tuesday we will see the radiologist and find out as much as we can about radiation.

Last night you told me that you were afraid of radiation because it might change you, the person you are, and your body. Especially since the oncologist told you that the hormones would change your body much more than radiation, both of us realize that it is not a rational fear. But it is your fear. As for me, that damned invisible duct tape has gotten tighter.

Hopefully, we will each sit down Sunday night and write out our questions for your Tuesday appointment. Maybe then we can compare questions and make only one list of them for the doctor. The oncologist suggested that maybe the radiologist would find a patient or two who could talk to you.

You and I are not aging well. Each time you have had something happen to you, you have moved more slowly. And Miriam once watched you as you were walking and noticed that you don't always pick up your feet. She felt you were a fall waiting to happen. She wasn't surprised when you fell shortly after. Once this prostate cancer is under control, I'm hoping that you will encourage your doctor to order physical therapy to strengthen your feet and legs as much as possible. Breast cancer be damned! I'm still hoping to be sitting on my balcony in a rocking chair when I am in my middle 90s and I'd like you to be with me!

Slowly we are putting together our minds and we're trying to plan ahead to make it easier to entertain ourselves once we find ourselves even less able to leave the apartment easily. The dog should help and having the DVD/CD player with our good TV will help. We can take trips on tape—seeing places we're not able to travel to. (Why do I think that doesn't appeal to you?)

I sometimes get scared of our future, but I'm also determined to do what I can to make me stronger and more useful. As you know, I've been practicing walking up stairs without my walker—getting ready for helping Phyllis who is 49 steps up. Well, I've walked 40 steps up—without stops—twice—and every day or so I will continue to walk steps. Since there are 16 steps between each floor in our building, I walk down first and then come back up and continue to the 3rd floor and up one more half level (8 steps). Yes, I'm winded, but it also feels good. By the time Phyllis gives birth, I intend to go all the way up to the 4th floor—48 steps. I have a goal of living long enough to laugh at the doctors. I have only 327 days until I retire—yahoo! The anticipation of retirement adds a delightful spoonful of whipped cream to my life. Meanwhile I will enjoy my life between now and then. Remember, I enjoy working with most of the people and I enjoy what I do. Then, on the personal side, we have 2 new grandbabies on the way this spring. Life is looking good. And I'm going to try to make it stay that way.

You and I will get through this prostate glitch Jay, and we will enjoy what we've got left. There are young people dying in wars and in big cities every day. Let's remember that we're the lucky ones. Yes, both of us have cancer and both of us have arthritis and the accompanying pain, but that doesn't mean life is over. We're just going to go on making our lives easier and more enjoyable. We've handled bumps in the road in the past and we will continue to do so and we're going to do it well.

Louise

May 21, 2008

My Dearest Louise,

This date of our marriage on May 21, 1976, it seems to be appropriate to let you know your light still shines on me. Technically your life ended with the third and final blow of cancer that invaded your lungs. This is not the end; I am still here today and will continue. I see the wonderful picture of both you and I with the love shining from our eyes—morning greeting: "Good morning, Louise. I love you." Evening, "Good night Louise. I love you."

The energy of your soul must be somewhere recharging with the thoughts of many who knew and were blessed by your love and caring.

I don't remember if I shared the following incident: Miriam came with the grand kids, Jacob and Selena for hello and visit at our condo unit. It was a warm summer day. Shoes (sandals) were as the custom, shed at the front door. This was a double occasion of joy for them to see and play with the newly obtained Maltese pup, Casey. Very soon, Selena squealed into Miriam's ear, "Mom, I stepped into Casey's pee." We laughed while we applied paper towels and sprayed the offending spot. Later, I thought what a grand moment—a circle of mother, daughter and granddaughter. This is a symbolic circle akin to our ring. Love is everywhere. Casey is 4 years old, showered by the custodian you left behind. He was your dog.

Love, Jay

P.S. I am following in your path of respect of humanity and a liberal application of good humor.

Eulogy for Louise Gordon by her son Michael Cohen

Louise Helen Roey Gordon was an amazing mother to Miriam, Phyllis and me. I wish that I could sufficiently articulate how much she loved us, how wonderful she was to us and how much we loved her.

Even though she accepted that life dealt some difficult blows to her, it pained her to see her children even slightly uncomfortable. On the flip side, she was so excited to hear about how we were happy. When I was living at home and went out at night, the hall light was left on. She could see the hall light from her bedroom, would wake-up at night, and be happy because she figured that I was out having fun. She figured that if I wasn't having fun, I would have come home.

She even loved us when we may have deserved it least. After I got suspended on the first day of high school because of a fight, she didn't berate me as one would expect. She knew how atypical it was for me and how upset I would be—so she had Phyllis go buy me an Izod shirt to cheer me up. She was able to figure out how we were feeling and tried to make us feel better.

You see, my mother derived immeasurable joy from her family—from her grandparents, her parents, her brother, her husband, her children, other relatives and most definitely from her grandchildren. The joy she felt being with Selena, Jacob, Alyssa and Eli radiated from her. The love she expressed when simply speaking to us emanated in her voice. She took such pleasure from learning that her children were spending time together. This showed her that the family bond she created was flourishing.

She cherished the strong friendships she created. She was a great listener and great support to so many people.

My mother enjoyed her brief retirement that she so greatly anticipated. But she also enjoyed her life throughout. She enjoyed not only the larger festive occasions but also the small facets of life. I recall driving down Lakeshore Drive and seeing how excited she was to see the skyline and the lake even though she already had seen them so many times. She created pleasure for herself by doing things like creating arts and crafts and by taking recorder lessons.

As you may have noticed I have used the words joy and pleasure a lot. This is because she created and viewed so many of her experiences as joyful and pleasurable.

There are many stories of my mother's spirit and positive attitude in the face of illness and great obstacles: from decorating her walker at festive occasions to refusing to feel sorry for herself. Her many physical limitations never stopped her from being active. She went out to dinner with friends, babysat, and got her weekly manicure. She also got her cherished puppy Casey just weeks ago.

One particular incident that stands out for me was a surgeon's response when I asked him to write a note to my mother's employer saying that she was well enough to work. He was shocked saying that he was prepared to write a letter saying that she was permanently disabled. He didn't understand who she was. Not only was she not going to limit herself by the term disabled, she deeply felt the importance of being alive. She was intent on not spending her time dying but intent on spending her time enjoying and living life. And live her life she did.

Memories of Louise Gordon

Louise Gordon was one of the most remarkable people I have ever known. She was intelligent, warm and caring—exuding incredible charm. Her inner strength and optimism were truly inspiring, but it was her attitude toward life which I admire most. All of the years that I knew her she faced significant health and familial challenges. Whenever I asked her about how things were going, she never sugarcoated her responses. She was a realist, but she also always expressed gratitude for the blessings she received. Pirkei Avot asks, "Who is rich?" and responds, "A person who is happy with her lot."

A person of lesser strength would have succumbed quickly to the physical and emotional assaults on her body and on her spirit, not Louise. She found ways to do much more than cope. She lived life with gusto. I will never forget when she was hospitalized with devastating back surgery, the result of her ongoing battles with cancer, and she could not have *seder* at home, how she arranged to have her family gather in her hospital room for *seder.*

She constantly worried about her children and her husband. In spite of her physical limitations she provided each of them with support, comfort and love. I do not think that I ever heard her happier than when she spoke about her grandchildren. To me, life seemed to be so unfair to Louise, but she always maintained that she had lived a good life. I never heard her complain. She had a sustaining faith, and her Judaism was part of her support system.

I still think of Louise every day as I drive to work or go out for my daily constitutional because I pass the complex where she and her beloved Jay lived. When I am tempted to complain about some problem or the vicissitudes of my life, I think of Louise and I count my blessings. I feel so fortunate to have known her and to have been her friend. She was one of those individuals who continue to inspire, even after they have died. Her memory is a blessing and her spirit still shines in the firmament of my daily existence. Louise Gordon defines what it meant to be a wealthy person and to leave a lasting legacy of love.

Rabbi Peter Knobel